Ketogenic Diet

Fat Bombs

Delicious Dessert Recipes that are High Fat and Low Carb for Weight Loss

Disclaimer

Copyright © 2016

All Rights Reserved.

No part of this eBook can be transmitted or reproduced in any form including print, electronic, photocopying, scanning, mechanical or recording without prior written permission from the author.

While the author has taken utmost efforts to ensure the accuracy of the written content, all readers are advised to follow information mentioned herein at their own risk. The author cannot be held responsible for any personal or commercial damage caused by information. All readers are encouraged to seek professional advice when needed.

About the Book

Does the idea of losing fat by eating fat sound ridiculous? Well, it is true! The Ketogenic diet is based on this theory. You can now indulge yourself in your most delightful treats that tickle your taste buds and satiate your cravings. Come fall in love with the sweet, creamy, crispy and melting textures of these delicious desserts. You can do this without having to worry about the calories that you are consuming. In fact, you would actually be losing weight all along! It can't get better than this, can it?

Before we get started with the recipes, it is important for you to understand what the Ketogenic diet is all about. To put it simply, this diet is a high fat and low carbohydrate based diet. You will simply be cutting down on the carbs instead of fat. You will have to make a few changes to your daily diet to get acclimatized to this diet. The positive results of this diet will start showing on your body within two weeks' time.

You can discover various tasty treats that will prove to be quite addictive. Welcome to the world of full fat cakes, pastries, cupcakes, muffins and other delicious desserts, so irresistible, that you will find yourself hurrying to the kitchen to cook! Let's sneak a peek at the mouthwatering treats that lie inside. Chocolate cakes, vanilla cheesecake, different varieties of cookies, muffins, chocolate bars, panna cottas, mousse and even popsicles!

I bet just the thought of these deserts is enough to get you hungry. Not only are these desserts delicious, but the detailed information rearing the serving size, prep-time, nutritional facts will definitely make it more appealing. The next time you have your friends and family over for a meal, you can proudly serve them the delicious and healthy treats that you have whipped up in your own kitchen. Wouldn't this make you feel proud and wonderful?

This book will change your perspective on dieting and a healthy lifestyle. Whoever said eating healthy doesn't mean eating anything tasty or sweet was obviously wrong!

Well, losing weight definitely doesn't get any yummier than this! So what are you waiting for?

About the Author

Sam Kuma is passionate about sharing his culinary experience to the world. His work involves modernization of healthy diet plans. He has published many recipe books for vegan, ketogenic, and paleo diets, dash food cooking, and several cookbooks on ethnic cuisines. His main focus is to make healthy diets like vegan and ketogenic mainstream by sharing easy-to-create, appetizing recipes. In his first two books regarding vegan recipes, he has produced delicious vegan chocolates, desserts, ice creams, burgers, and sandwiches.

Table of Contents

Disclaimer 2

About the Book 4

About the Author 7

Table of Contents 9

Introduction 13

Tiramisu Icecream Fat Bombs 16

White Chocolate Butter Pecan Fat Bombs 19

Mint and Chocolate Chip Icecream Fat Bombs 21

Strawberry Basil Ice Cups 23

Peanut Butter Cups 25

Chocolate Mudslide 26

Blackberry Cheesecake Bombs 28

Strawberry Cheesecake Fat Bombs 30

Blueberry Cheesecake Popsicles 32

Pumpkin Cheesecake Fat Bombs 34

Peanut Butter Mousse 37

Blueberry Mousse 38

Lime Mousse Fat Bomb 40

Dark Chocolate Fat Bomb Mousse 42

Chocolate Peanut Butter Dream Cream 44

Raspberry Ice Cream Fat Bomb 46

Mocha Ice Cream Fat Bomb 48

Blueberry Ice Cream Fat Bomb 50

Strawberry Swirl Ice Cream Fat Bomb 52

Chocolate Peanut Butter Bombs 55

Chocolate Chip Peanut Butter Ice cream 57

Coeur a la Crème 60

Apple-Apricot Cloud 64

Cream Cheese Clouds 66

Keto Nutella Bombs 67

Creamy Peanut Butter Dessert 70

Raspberry Panna Cotta 72

Chocolate Chip Pudding Fat Bomb 74

Lemon Cheesecake Pudding Fat Bomb 75

Vanilla Crème Pudding Parfaits..................................... 76

Blueberry Fat Bombs 78

Butter Fat Bombs 80

Energy Fat Bars... 83

Chocolate Coconut Candies... 86

No Bake Chocolate Peanut Butter Truffles 89

No Bake Raspberry Cheesecake Truffles 91

Sesame and Coconut Fat Bombs................................... 93

Chocolate Almond Fat Bomb 96

Almond Butter Bombs 98

Peppermint Fat Bombs... 100

Coconut Fat Bombs... 102

Easter Egg Fat Bombs... 103

Coconut and Cinnamon Fat Bombs 106

Vanilla Fat Bomb... 108

Fudgy Macadamia Chocolate Fat Bombs 110

Cinnamon Bun Fat Bomb Bars 112

Chocolate Raspberry Fat Bombs 114

Chocolate Almond Fat Bomb 116

Stacked Choco-nut Bombs.. 118

Chocolate Fat Bombs 120

Valentine Day Treat 122

Coconut Chocolate Fat Bombs 124

Easy Lemon Fat Bombs 126

Caramel Apple Pie Fat Bomb 128

Pumpkin Pie Fat Bombs.. 130

Orange & Walnut Chocolate Fat Bombs 133

Keto Mounds Fat Bombs 135

Orange Butter Pecan Fat Bombs.................................. 138

Conclusion 140

Introduction

I want to thank you for downloading this book "Ketogenic Diet: Fat Bombs- Delicious Dessert Recipes that are High Fat and Low Carb for Weight Loss".

Most Ketogenic recipe books tend to steer clear of the sweet stuff leading to a plate of bland meat that isn't appealing. The problem with such diets is that you might end up craving for something sweet in between meals. Fat bombs are the perfect solution to your problems.

Fat bombs are nothing but a healthy combination of foods that are rich in fat and create an explosion of nutritious flavor. This is a healthy way to fuel your body through this diet while satiating your cravings for something sweet.

When you are consuming a fat bomb, there are certain benefits that you experience. The process of fat loss is accelerated, you will find a surge in your energy levels and feel more vitalized, you will be able to control your appetite, your hormones would be thoroughly balanced and your blood sugar levels will be low. This also lowers your cholesterol. Another important benefit of munching on these Ketogenic desserts is that your mental focus improves.

All the recipes given in this book have been developed keeping in mind the requirements of the Ketogenic diet. The recipes have been tried and tested. The results have always been surprisingly good. You will not only be able to sneak in a sweet treat when you crave for one, but you will not be putting on any extra weight while doing so. In fact, you will be shedding those extra kilos.

Before we get started, you will need to understand that if you are serious about shedding those extra kilos then you will have to commit yourself to the Ketogenic diet. You will need to eat and avoid certain things and you shouldn't sneak in any cheat snacks. A little bit of commitment and extra effort will definitely go a long way, especially when it comes to making yourself healthier?

Following a diet couldn't have been more fun!

So, let's get started!

Tiramisu Icecream Fat Bombs

| Prep: 10 min | Total: 20 min + freezing time | Serving: 6 |

Ingredients:

For the ice bombs:

- 2/3 cup mascarpone cheese (you can alternatively use creamed coconut milk)
- 2 tablespoons strong brewed coffee, chilled
- 2 tablespoons Swerve or powdered erythritol
- Liquid stevia drops to taste
- 1 teaspoon rum extract (opt for sugar free)

For the coating

- 0.5-ounce cacao butter
- 0.7 ounce 90% dark chocolate

Instructions:

1. Add mascarpone cheese, erythritol, rum extract and coffee to the mixing bowl. Beat with an electric mixer until smooth and creamy.
2. Add stevia and beat again.
3. Add about 2 tablespoons of the mixture into circular molds or small silicone muffin molds.
4. Freeze until set.
5. Meanwhile, add dark chocolate and cacao butter to a bowl and melt either in a microwave or in a double boiler. Cool for a while.
6. Remove from the freezer. Thread a frozen bomb into a toothpick and immediately dip into the

melted chocolate. Coat well. Place on a lined freezer safe dish.

7. Freeze again until the chocolate coating hardens.

White Chocolate Butter Pecan Fat Bombs

| Prep: 15 min | Total: 50 min | Serving: 8 |

Ingredients:

- 4 tablespoons butter
- 4 tablespoons coconut oil
- 1 cup pecans or walnuts or hazelnuts, chopped
- 4 ounces' cocoa butter
- 1/2 teaspoon vanilla extract
- 4 tablespoons powdered erythritol
- A large pinch salt
- A large pinch stevia

Instructions:

1. Add butter, coconut oil and cocoa butter to a small pan and place over low heat.

2. When the ingredients are melted, remove from heat.
3. Add vanilla, salt, and stevia and stir.
4. Take 8 silicone cupcake molds or candy molds. Drop a few pieces of pecans in each.
5. Pour the mixture into each mold.
6. Freeze for 30 minutes or until set and serve.

Mint and Chocolate Chip Ice-cream Fat Bombs

Prep: 7 min	Total: 10 min + freezing time	Serving: 7

Ingredients:

- 1/2 cup full fat mascarpone cheese or creamed coconut milk
- 1 ounce 90 % dark chocolate, chopped
- 2 1/2 tablespoons powdered erythritol or Swerve
- Liquid stevia drops to taste (optional)
- 1/2 teaspoon peppermint extract or 2 teaspoons fresh mint, minced

Instructions:

1. Add all the ingredients to a blender and blend until smooth. Transfer into a bowl.
2. Add about 2 tablespoons of the mixture into circular molds or small silicone muffin molds.
3. Freeze until set.

Strawberry Basil Ice Cups

| Prep: 5 min | Total: 15 min + freezing time | Serving: 5 |

Ingredients:

- 6 tablespoons cream cheese
- 4 tablespoons creamed coconut milk
- 2 tablespoons butter, unsalted, at room temperature
- 2 tablespoons powdered erythritol or Swerve
- Liquid stevia drops to taste (optional)
- A handful fresh basil leaves
- 1/2 cup fresh strawberries + extra to garnish
- 1/2 teaspoon vanilla extract

Instructions:

1. Add all the ingredients (except strawberries and basil) to a blender and blend until smooth.
2. Remove half the blended mixture and set aside.
3. To the other half that is in the blender add strawberries and blend until smooth.
4. Divide the mixture into 5 silicone muffin cups.
5. Clean the blender and add the blended mixture that was set aside. Add basil leaves and blend until smooth.
6. Divide the mixture and spoon into the muffin cups above the strawberry layer.
7. Place thinly sliced strawberry slices on top.
8. Freeze for a few hours until set.

Peanut Butter Cups

Prep: 5 min	Total: 15 min + freezing time	Serving: 6

Ingredients:

- 2 cup heavy whipping cream
- 1 cup peanut butter
- Stevia sweetened chocolate syrup to drizzle

Instructions:

1. Whip together peanut butter and whipping cream.
2. Line muffin tins with cupcake papers.
3. Fill the muffin tin with the whipped mixture. Drizzle chocolate syrup over it.
4. Freeze until set and serve.

Chocolate Mudslide

Prep: 5 min	Total: 10 min + freezing time	Serving: 6

Ingredients:

- 2 cups heavy cream
- 6 tablespoons cocoa, unsweetened
- 1 cup stevia sweetened chocolate syrup
- 1 cup water
- 2 teaspoons vanilla extract

Instructions:

1. Place a saucepan over medium heat. Add all the ingredients except vanilla and bring to the boil.

2. Lower heat and simmer for 5 minutes. Stir occasionally.
3. Remove from heat. Add vanilla and stir. Cool completely.
4. Pour into ice trays and freeze.

Blackberry Cheesecake Bombs

Prep: 10 min	Total: 15 min + chilling time	Serving: 6

Ingredients:

- 1 cup cream cheese, softened
- 1/2 cup heavy cream
- 4 eggs
- 2 teaspoons lemon juice
- 1 teaspoon vanilla extract
- Sugar substitute like stevia to taste
- 1 cup frozen blackberries, thawed
- 1/2 cup fresh blackberries

- Whipped cream to serve

Instructions:

1. Place cream cheese, heavy cream, eggs, lemon juice, vanilla extract, stevia and frozen blackberries in a microwave safe bowl. Whisk well until smooth.
2. Microwave on high for 90 seconds stirring in between.
3. Pour into individual muffin cups. Cool.
4. Chill until set.
5. Serve with fresh blackberries and whipped cream.

Strawberry Cheesecake Fat Bombs

| Prep: 5 min | Total: 10 min + chilling time | Serving: 5 |

Ingredients:

- 1 1/2 cups cream cheese, at room temperature
- 1 cup strawberries, fresh or frozen
- Strawberry slices for garnish
- 1/2 cup butter, chopped into small pieces, softened
- 1 tablespoon vanilla extract
- 30 drops liquid stevia or 4 tablespoons erythritol

Instructions:

1. Add softened butter and cream cheese to a bowl and mix until well combined.

2. Add the strawberries, vanilla and stevia to a blender and blend until smooth. Transfer into the bowl of cream cheese. Whisk well.
3. Transfer the mixture into candy molds or small muffin molds.
4. Chill until set and serve.

Blueberry Cheesecake Popsicles

| Prep: 5 min | Total: 10 min + chilling time | Serving: 5 |

Ingredients:

- 1 cup cream cheese
- 4 cups fresh blueberries
- 6 tablespoons erythritol or Sweetener or to taste
- 4 cups heavy whipped cream.

Instructions:

1. Add all the ingredients except cream to a blender and blend until smooth.
2. Transfer into a bowl. Add cream and fold gently.
3. Pour into Popsicle molds and freeze until done.

4. Remove the molds from the freezer 10 minutes before serving. Invert on to a plate and serve.
5. Alternately, you can pour in the ice cube trays and freeze.

Pumpkin Cheesecake Fat Bombs

Prep: 5 min	Total: 10 min + chilling time	Serving: 5

Ingredients:

- 6 ounces' cream cheese
- 1 cup butter, unsalted
- 1/2 cup pecans, chopped + extra for topping
- 1 cup pumpkin puree
- 1 1/2 tablespoons vanilla extract
- 8 tablespoons truvia or erythritol or to taste
- 2 teaspoons ground cinnamon
- 1/4 teaspoon salt
- 1 teaspoon pumpkin pie spice

Instructions:

1. Line a pie pan with wax paper.
2. Place a saucepan over medium high heat. Add butter. Stir and let the butter melt.
3. Add pumpkin puree and continue stirring.
4. Add rest of the ingredients (except vanilla extract) and whisk until smooth.
5. Add vanilla extract and stir until well combined.
6. Remove from heat. Pour the mixture into the lined pie pan.
7. Sprinkle pecans over it.
8. Place in the freezer for at least 8 hours.
9. Remove from the freezer and discard the wax paper.
10. Chop into squares.

11. Serve. The unused ones can be placed in an airtight container. Freeze the container until use.

Peanut Butter Mousse

Prep: 5 min	Total: 10 min + chilling time	Serving: 6

Ingredients:

- 3 tablespoons peanut butter
- 3/4 cup heavy cream
- 1 1/2 cups raspberries

Instructions:

1. Blend together all the ingredients in a blender until smooth. Transfer into a bowl.
2. Alternately, you can pour into small silicone muffin moulds.
3. Chill and serve later.

Blueberry Mousse

Prep: 5 min	Total: 10 min + chilling time	Serving: 12 - 14

Ingredients:

- 3 cups blueberries
- 2 cups firm tofu, drained, crumbled
- 1 cup mascarpone cheese
- 1 cup heavy cream
- 5 tablespoons erythritol or Swerve sweetener
- Dark dairy-free chocolate, shaved to serve

Instructions:

1. Add blueberries to the blender and blend.

2. Add tofu and blend until smooth. Add sweetener, mascarpone cheese, and cream. Blend until well combined.
3. Transfer into individual serving bowls. Refrigerate for 3-4 hours before serving.
4. Serve garnished with chocolate shavings and a few blueberries.

Lime Mousse Fat Bomb

Prep: 5 min	Total: 15 min + chilling time	Serving: 8

Ingredients:

- 2 cups heavy cream
- 4 ounces' cream cheese
- 7-8 tablespoons erythritol or Swerve sweetener or to taste
- 2 teaspoons coconut extract or vanilla extract
- 1/2 cup fresh lime juice
- Coconut flakes to garnish, unsweetened (optional)

Instructions:

1. Add cream cheese to the mixing bowl and beat with an electric mixer until smooth and creamy.
2. Add erythritol and beat until well blended. Add lime juice and beat again.
3. Add coconut extract and heavy cream and beat until well blended
4. Transfer into individual 8 dessert bowls.
5. Garnish with coconut flakes.
6. Chill and serve later.

Dark Chocolate Fat Bomb Mousse

Prep: 5 min	Total: 15 min + chilling time	Serving: 6

Ingredients:

- 4 ounces' cream cheese, softened
- 4 ounces' butter, unsalted
- 6 ounces' heavy cream, whipped
- 2 tablespoons erythritol or Swerve sweetener
- 2 tablespoons cocoa powder, unsweetened

Instructions:

1. Add butter and erythritol to the mixing bowl and beat with an electric mixer until smooth.

2. Add cream cheese and beat until well blended.

   Add cocoa and beat until smooth.

3. Add whipped cream and mix well.

4. Transfer into 6 silicone moulds and chill.

Chocolate Peanut Butter Dream Cream

Prep: 10 min	Total: 15 min + freezing time	Serving: 8

Ingredients:

- 3 large Hass avocados, peeled, pitted, chopped
- 1/2 cup peanut butter, unsweetened
- 1/2 cup mascarpone cheese
- 1/2 cup cocoa powder
- 20 drops liquid stevia or to taste (optional)

Instructions:

1. Blend together all the ingredients with the peanut butter until smooth and creamy.

2. Line muffin tins with cupcake papers. Pour into the lined muffin tins.
3. Freeze until done.
4. Remove from the freezer 15 minutes before serving.
5. Scoop and serve.
6. You can also serve it chilled if you do not like it frozen.

Raspberry Ice Cream Fat Bomb

Prep: 5 min	Total: 7 min + freezing time	Serving: 6

Ingredients:

- 3 cups heavy whipping cream
- 1 1/2 cups raspberries + extra for garnishing
- Few drops of stevia sweetener or any other sweetener of your choice (optional)

Instructions:

1. Add all the ingredients to a blender. Blend until smooth.
2. Freeze the ice cream for 5-6 hours or until set.

3. Remove from the freezer around 30 minutes before serving.

4. Scoop into dessert bowls.

5. Garnish with raspberries and serve.

Mocha Ice Cream Fat Bomb

Prep: 2 min	Total: 5 min + freezing time	Serving: 6

Ingredients:

- 2 cups coconut milk
- 1 cup heavy cream
- 1/4 cup Erythritol
- 30 drops liquid stevia
- 1/4 cup cocoa powder
- 2 tablespoons instant coffee
- 1/2 teaspoon. Xanthan Gum

Instructions:

1. Mix together all the ingredients (except xanthan gum) in a mixing bowl. With a stick blender, blend the ingredients.
2. Add the xanthan gum little by little, blending continuously.
3. Freeze the ice cream for 5-6 hours or until set. Remove from the freezer around 30 minutes before serving.
4. Scoop into dessert bowls.
5. Serve sprinkled with a little instant coffee.

Blueberry Ice Cream Fat Bomb

Prep: 2 min	Total: 10 min + freezing time	Serving: 6

Ingredients:

- 3/4 cup crème Fraiche
- 3/4 cup blueberries, fresh or frozen
- 1 1/2 cups heavy cream
- 1 tablespoon vanilla protein powder
- 2 yolks

Instructions:

1. Whip cream in a bowl until slightly fluffy.
2. Whip crème Fraiche in another larger bowl until slightly fluffy.

3. Add most of the whipped cream to it. Also add yolk, and most of the blueberries and whip well.
4. Freeze for an hour or until set.
5. Scoop into individual dessert bowls. Dot with remaining whipped cream and sprinkle the remaining blueberries and serve.

Strawberry Swirl Ice Cream Fat Bomb

Prep: 5 min	Total: 30 min + freezing time	Serving: 12

Ingredients:

For vanilla ice cream:

- 2 cups heavy cream
- 2 tablespoons vodka (optional)
- 6 large egg yolks
- 2/3 cup erythritol
- 1/4 teaspoon xanthan gum (optional)
- 1 teaspoon vanilla extract

For strawberry swirl ice cream:

- 2 cups strawberries, pureed

Instructions:

1. Place a heavy bottomed pan over low heat. Add cream and erythritol. Heat until erythritol dissolves. Remove from heat.
2. Add eggs to the mixing bowl and beat with an electric mixer until it doubles in volume.
3. Add about 2 tablespoons of the warm cream to the egg and beat constantly. Repeat this procedure until all the cream is added. Add vanilla and beat again.
4. Add vodka and xanthan gum and beat again. Cool completely.
5. Freeze the ice cream for a couple of hours. Stir in between a couple of times while it is being frozen.

6. Remove the semi-frozen ice cream from the freezer.
7. Swirl the strawberry puree all around on the top. With a knife, lightly mix to get a ripple effect.
8. Freeze the ice cream for another 5-6 hours or until set. Remove from the freezer around 30 minutes before serving.
9. Scoop and serve.
10. For making vanilla ice cream fat bomb, omit steps 6 and 7. Freeze until set.

Chocolate Peanut Butter Bombs

Prep: 10 min	Total: 15 min + freezing time	Serving: 8

Ingredients:

- 4 large Hass avocados, peeled, pitted, chopped
- 1/2 cup peanut butter, unsweetened
- 1/2 cup cocoa powder
- 20 drops liquid stevia or to taste (optional)

Instructions:

1. Blend together all the ingredients except peanut butter until smooth and creamy.
2. Pour into a freezer safe container. Add peanut butter. With a knife, swirl the peanut butter.

3. Freeze until done.

4. Remove from the freezer 15 minutes before serving.

5. Scoop and serve in individual dessert bowls

Chocolate Chip Peanut Butter Ice cream

| Prep: 10 min | Total: 30 min | Serving: 10 |

Ingredients:

- 1 cup almond milk
- 1 cup heavy cream
- 2 tablespoons vodka (optional)
- 6 large egg yolks
- 1/2 cup erythritol
- 1/4 teaspoon xanthan gum (optional)
- 2 teaspoons vanilla extract
- 1 cup peanut butter
- 1 1/2 cups sugar-free chocolate chips

Instructions:

1. Place a heavy bottomed pan over low heat. Add milk, cream, and erythritol. Heat until erythritol dissolves. Remove from heat.
2. Add eggs to the mixing bowl and beat with an electric mixer until it doubles in volume.
3. Add about 2 tablespoons of the warm cream to the egg and beat constantly. Repeat this procedure until all the cream is added. Add vanilla and beat again.
4. Add vodka and xanthan gum and beat again. Cool completely.
5. Freeze the ice cream for a couple of hours. Stir in between a couple of times while it is being frozen.

6. Remove the semi-frozen ice cream from the freezer.
7. Add chocolate chips and whisk well. Add peanut butter and fold lightly.
8. Freeze the ice cream for another 5-6 hours or until set. Remove from the freezer around 30 minutes before serving.
9. Scoop and serve.

Coeur a la Crème

Prep: 15 min	Total: 35 minutes + chilling time	Serving: 12

Ingredients:

- 1 cup heavy cream
- 8 ounces' cream cheese
- 1/2 cup sour cream, cultured
- 1/2 cup small curd cottage cheese
- 3 tablespoons erythritol or Swerve sweetener
- 1/4 teaspoon salt
- 2 teaspoons vanilla extract

To serve:

- 1 cup strawberries, sliced

- 2 tablespoons erythritol

Instructions:

1. Take 8 Coeur la crème molds of about 3-4 inches' size (heart shaped molds)
2. Take 8 square pieces of cheesecloth, the size of about 10 x 10 inches.
3. Dip the pieces of cloth in water and remove it immediately. Squeeze the cloth of water. It should be moist.
4. Line the molds with this cheesecloth. The remaining cloth should fall out of the mold.
5. To make Coeur: Add cream cheese, cottage cheese, and sour cream to a food processor and pulse until smooth and creamy.
6. Transfer into a bowl.

7. Add cream, erythritol, vanilla and salt to a bowl and beat with an electric mixer.
8. Beat until stiff peaks are formed.
9. Add this into the bowl of cream cheese and fold gently. Spoon into the molds. Cover the molds with the part of the cloth that is falling out of the mold.
10. Place the filled molds in a shallow baking dish.
11. Chill for at least 5-6 hours.
12. Meanwhile, add erythritol to strawberries and stir to lightly mash it. Set aside for a while.
13. Unwrap the cloth and invert onto a plate.
14. Spoon some sweetened strawberries on top and serve.

Apple-Apricot Cloud

Prep: 5 min	Total: 15 min + chilling time	Serving: 20

Ingredients:

- 32 ounces' apple-apricot sauce, unsweetened
- 3 cups heavy cream
- 4 tablespoons erythritol or Swerve sweetener

Instructions:

1. Add cream and erythritol to the mixing bowl and beat with an electric mixer until firm peaks are formed.
2. Add apple-apricot sauce and fold gently.

3. Line a baking sheet with wax paper. Drop spoonfuls on the baking sheet.

4. Chill and serve later.

Cream Cheese Clouds

Prep: 5 min	Total: 15 min + chilling time	Serving: 12

Ingredients:

- 1/4 cup butter, unsalted, softened
- 4 ounces' cream cheese, softened
- 1/4 teaspoon vanilla extract
- 1/4 cup granular Splenda or erythritol

Instructions:

1. Add cream and Splenda to the mixing bowl and beat with an electric mixer until firm peaks are formed.
2. Drop spoonfuls in a square mold.
3. Chill and serve later.

Keto Nutella Bombs

Prep: 10 min	Total: 55 min + chilling time	Serving: 24

Ingredients:

- 4 cups hazelnuts
- 1 cup erythritol
- 1/2 cup cocoa powder, unsweetened
- 1/2 cup heavy cream
- 1/2 teaspoons salt
- 2 tablespoons coconut oil or butter
- 1/2 cup water
- 2 teaspoons vanilla extract

Instructions:

1. Spread the hazelnuts on a baking sheet in a single layer.
2. Bake in a preheated oven 425°F for about 12 -15 minutes or until brown (The skin will be nearly dark brown when done).
3. Remove from the oven and cool.
4. Spread a moist kitchen towel on your work area. Spread the roasted hazelnuts on one-half of the towel. Cover with the other half of the towel and rub for a while until the skin peels off.
5. Transfer the hazelnuts to your food processor and pulse for a couple of minutes. It should be of peanut butter consistency.
6. Add rest of the ingredients and blend until smooth.

7. Line muffin tins with cupcake paper. Spoon in about 2 tablespoons of Nutella into each.

8. Chill and serve.

Creamy Peanut Butter Dessert

| Prep: 5 min | Total: 10 min + chilling time | Serving: 4 |

Ingredients:

- 6 tablespoons peanut butter, unsalted
- Sweetener of your choice
- 1/2 cup whipped cream
- 1 tablespoon cocoa powder

Instructions:

1. Divide the peanut butter and place into 4 individual muffin cups (about 1 1/2 tablespoons)
2. Sprinkle sweetener over it.
3. Spread some cream over the peanut butter.

4. Sprinkle cocoa powder over the cream.

5. Divide the remaining cream (if it is remaining) amongst the bowls.

6. Chill and serve later.

Raspberry Panna Cotta

| Prep: 10 min | Total: 20 min + chilling time | Serving: 8 |

Ingredients:

- 2 cups almond milk, unsweetened
- 2 cups heavy cream
- 2 sachets unflavored gelatin
- 1/2 cup erythritol or Swerve sweetener
- 1 cup sugar-free raspberry jam
- 2 tablespoons fresh lemon juice
- 2 teaspoons vanilla extract
- Raspberries to garnish

Instructions:

1. Place a saucepan over low heat. Add heavy cream and almond milk and stir.
2. Add erythritol and gelatin and heat until the mixture is warm. Do not boil. Whisk until the sweetener is dissolved.
3. Remove from heat. Add vanilla and lemon juice and stir. Pour into 8 greased ramekins.
4. Cover with cling film and chill for at least 4-5 hours.
5. To serve: Run a knife all around the edges of the pannacotta and invert onto a plate.
6. Slice and serve garnished with raspberries.

Chocolate Chip Pudding Fat Bomb

| Prep: 5 min | Total: 10 min + chilling time | Serving: 6 |

Ingredients:

- 16 ounces' cream cheese, softened
- 8 ounces heavy whipping cream
- 8-10 drops liquid stevia or any other artificial sweetener to taste
- 2 ounces' dark chocolate, finely chopped

Instructions:

1. Whisk together all the ingredients until smooth.
2. Pour into individual dessert bowls.
3. Chill until set and serve later.

Lemon Cheesecake Pudding Fat Bomb

Prep: 2 min	Total: 5 min + chilling time	Serving: 4

Ingredients:

- 12 ounces of softened cream cheese
- 3/4 cup heavy cream
- 6-7 packets of artificial sweetener
- 1 teaspoon lemon extract

Instructions:

1. Blend together all the ingredients until smooth and pour into individual dessert bowls.
2. Chill and serve later.

Vanilla Crème Pudding Parfaits

Prep: 10 min	Total: 17 min + chilling time	Serving: 8

Ingredients:

- 2 cans (14.5 ounces each) full-fat coconut milk, chilled
- 2 teaspoons vanilla extract
- 20 drops liquid stevia
- 1/2 cup walnuts, chopped
- 1 1/2 cups fresh berries of your choice
- Ground cinnamon to garnish

Instructions:

1. To make vanilla crème: Pour coconut milk into the bowl of your stand mixer. Add stevia and vanilla extract. Whisk until well combined.

2. Add berries and walnuts to a bowl. Toss well.
3. Take 8 parfait glasses. Add about 3 spoonfuls of vanilla crème into each of the glasses.
4. Use about 1/2 of the berry mixture and layer over the vanilla crème.
5. Next layer with the remaining vanilla crème followed by the remaining half of the berry mixture.
6. Sprinkle ground cinnamon on top
7. Chill and serve.

Blueberry Fat Bombs

| Prep: 10 min | Total: 17 min + chilling time | Serving: 8 |

Ingredients:

- 1 3/4 cups blueberries
- 1 1/4 cup coconut oil
- 8 ounces' butter
- 1/2 cup coconut cream
- 8 ounces' cream cheese, softened, at room temperature
- Stevia or erythritol to taste

Instructions:

1. Add all the ingredients to a blender and blend until the consistency you desire is achieved.
2. Place silicone candy molds on a baking sheet. Pour the blended mixture into the tray.
3. Freeze until set.
4. Remove it from the molds and serve.

Butter Fat Bombs

Prep: 5 min	Total: 17 min + chilling time	Serving: 12

Ingredients:

- 2 sticks butter
- 16 ounces' raw coconut butter
- 16 ounces' almond butter
- 2 bars 85% dark chocolate chips or chocolate
- 4 tablespoons butter for ganache
- 4 tablespoons erythritol or to taste (optional)
- Roasted nuts (optional)
- Dried cranberries or any other low carb dried fruit

Instructions:

1. Add butter stick, almond butter and coconut butter to a microwave safe bowl.
2. Microwave on high for a couple of minutes until melted.
3. Remove from the microwave and stir until well combined. Add sweetener if using and stir.
4. Pour the mixture into small muffin cups or chocolate molds.
5. Cool completely and chill until hardened.
6. Meanwhile make ganache as follows: Add chocolate and 4 tablespoons butter to a microwave safe bowl.
7. Microwave for about a minute or until melted. Remove from the microwave and mix. Let it cool for a few minutes.

8. Remove the chilled bombs from the refrigerator.

9. Line a baking sheet with wax paper.

10. Dip the chilled bomb in the melted chocolate and place on the baking sheet.

11. Chill until the chocolate hardens and serve.

Energy Fat Bars

Prep: 10 min	Total: 15 min + chilling time	Serving: 12

Ingredients:

- 4 tablespoons coconut flour
- 6 tablespoons black chia seeds, lightly toasted
- 1 cup coconut flakes, unsweetened
- 3/4 cup heavy whipping cream, divided
- 4 tablespoons almond butter or any other nut butter of your choice
- 2 tablespoons erythritol or any other sweetener to taste
- 1/2 teaspoon maple flavoring

- 2 tablespoons MCT oil
- 1 teaspoon pumpkin pie spice

Instructions:

1. Place a saucepan over medium heat. Add 1/2-cup cream and erythritol and stir. Heat until bubbly and remove from heat. Set aside to cool for 10 minutes.
2. Add almond butter, oil, 2 tablespoons cream, maple flavoring, and pumpkin pie spice. Mix well.
3. Place a pan over medium heat. Add chia seeds, coconut flakes and coconut flour and toast until it just begins to turn golden brown in color.
4. Remove from heat. Transfer into the pan of cream. Add the remaining cream and stir.

5. Transfer onto a lined baking sheet. Chill for about 30 minutes or until set.

6. Chop into rectangles and serve.

Chocolate Coconut Candies

Prep: 10 min	Total: 15 min + chilling time	Serving: 10 mini cups

Ingredients:

For coconut candies:

- 1/4 cup coconut oil
- 1/4 cup shredded coconut, unsweetened
- 1/4 cup coconut butter
- 1 1/2 tablespoons Swerve sweetener or any other sweetener of your choice

For chocolate topping:

- 0.5-ounce chocolate, unsweetened
- 0.75-ounce cocoa butter
- 2 tablespoons cocoa powder, unsweetened
- 2 tablespoons Swerve sweetener

- 1/4 teaspoon vanilla extract

Instructions:

1. Line mini muffin pans with mini parchment liners.
2. Add coconut oil and coconut butter to a small saucepan. Place the saucepan over low heat to melt. Stir.
3. Add shredded coconut and sweetener and mix well.
4. Pour into the muffin pan.
5. Freeze for about 30 minutes or until firm.
6. For chocolate topping: Place cocoa butter and chocolate in a heatproof bowl. Place the bowl on a double boiler and heat until the chocolate is melted.
7. Add sweetener and cocoa and mix well.

8. Remove from heat. Let it cool for 5 minutes. Add vanilla and stir.

9. Pour over the chilled coconut cups.

10. Chill again until it hardens and serve.

No Bake Chocolate Peanut Butter Truffles

| Prep: 5 min | Total: 2 hrs. | Serving: 6 |

Ingredients:

- 2 tablespoons butter, melted
- 1/2 cup peanut butter
- 3 ounces' sugar-free chocolate chips
- 3/4 cup powdered erythritol

Instructions:

1. Add peanut butter, butter and erythritol to a bowl and mix well. If you find the mixture too watery, refrigerate for 30 minutes.
2. Divide the mixture into 6 parts and shape each part into balls. Place on a lined baking sheet.

3. Chill for about 45 minutes.
4. Meanwhile, place chocolate chips in a microwave-safe bowl and microwave until melted.
5. Now dip the balls into the melted chocolate. Remove with a slotted spoon and place it back on the lined baking sheet.
6. Chill until the chocolate coating is hardened and serve.

No Bake Raspberry Cheesecake Truffles

| Prep: 5 min | Total: 3 hrs. | Serving: 8 |

Ingredients:

- 4 ounces' cream cheese, softened, at room temperature
- 1 tablespoon heavy cream
- 2 tablespoons coconut oil, melted
- 1/4 cup Swerve sweetener or erythritol
- 1/2 teaspoon vanilla flavored stevia
- 1 1/2 teaspoons raspberry extract
- 3/4 cup sugar-free chocolate chips, melted
- A few drops red food coloring

Instructions:

1. Add cream cheese and sweetener to the mixing bowl and beat with an electric mixer until smooth.
2. Add cream, stevia, salt, raspberry extract, and food coloring and beat again
3. Add oil and blend until well combined. Place the bowl in the refrigerator and chill for an hour.
4. Line a baking sheet with wax paper. Drop spoonfuls or mini cookie scoops of the mixture on the baking sheet. This should make around 24 balls.
5. Freeze for about an hour.
6. Dip the frozen balls in melted chocolate. Place on the baking sheet.
7. Chill until the chocolate hardens and serve.

Sesame and Coconut Fat Bombs

Prep: 5 min	Total: 30 min + chilling time	Serving: 16 fat bombs

Ingredients:

For the truffles:

- 1/2 cup coconut butter
- 1/2 cup firm coconut oil, chilled if necessary
- 1/4 cup full-fat coconut milk, chilled overnight
- 1/8 teaspoon ground cinnamon
- 1/4 teaspoon matcha green tea powder
- 1/2 teaspoon vanilla extract
- 1/8 teaspoon Himalayan salt

For the coating:

- 1/2 tablespoon Sesame seeds
- 1/2 cup finely shredded coconut, unsweetened
- ¼ cup poppy seeds

Instructions:

1. To make truffles: Add all the ingredients of the truffle to a mixing bowl. Beat with an electric mixer until light and creamy.
2. Chill for an hour.
3. Meanwhile, mix together the coating ingredients in a bowl.
4. Remove the chilled mixture. Take out 16 small scoops of the mixture using small ice cream scoop.
5. Roll the scoops into a round shape. Dredge the balls in the coating mixture and place in an airtight container. Chill until use.

6. Remove from the refrigerator about 15 minutes before eating.

Chocolate Almond Fat Bomb

Prep: 5 min	Total: 20 min + chilling time	Serving: 25 fat bombs

Ingredients:

- 2 cups coconut oil
- 25 whole almonds
- 2 cups almond butter
- 1/2 coconut flour
- 1 cup cocoa powder, unsweetened
- Stevia drops to taste

Instructions:

1. Place a saucepan over medium heat. Add almond butter and coconut oil. Heat until it melts. Stir and add rest of the ingredients.
2. Remove from heat and cool.
3. Divide into 25 portions.
4. Place an almond in each portion in the center and shape into balls.
5. Chill and serve.

Almond Butter Bombs

Prep: 5 min	Total: 15 min + freezing time	Serving: 10 fat bombs

Ingredients:

- 4 tablespoons almond butter
- 4 tablespoons coconut oil
- 1/2 teaspoon ground cinnamon
- Erythritol or Swerve sweetener to taste

Instructions:

1. Place all the ingredients in a heatproof bowl.
2. Place the bowl in a double boiler and heat until melted.
3. Pour into 10 silicone molds or make circular bars of the same.

4. Freeze and serve.

Peppermint Fat Bombs

| Prep: 5 min | Total: 15 min + chilling time | Serving: 12 fat bombs |

Ingredients:

- 4 tablespoons cocoa powder, unsweetened
- 9 ounces' coconut oil, melted
- 1/2 teaspoon peppermint extract
- 2 tablespoons granulated erythritol or Swerve sweetener

Instructions:

1. Mix together oil, sweetener and peppermint extract.

2. Set aside half of this mixture.

3. Pour the other half into 12 small silicone moulds. Chill until it hardens.

4. Add cocoa powder to the mixture that was set aside.

5. Remove the molds from the refrigerator. Pour the cocoa mixture over it.

6. Chill until it hardens and serve.

Coconut Fat Bombs

| Prep: 5 min | Total: 10 min + chilling time | Serving: 20 fat bombs |

Ingredients:

- 5.2 ounces' coconut oil, melted
- 5.2 ounces' coconut butter, softened,
- 3 teaspoons powdered erythritol or Swerve sweetener or to taste
- 1.6 ounces finely shredded coconut

Instructions:

1. Add all the ingredients to a bowl and mix well.
2. Transfer into ice cube trays or 20 small silicone moulds.
3. Chill and serve.

Easter Egg Fat Bombs

| Prep: 30 min | Total: 50 min + chilling time | Serving: 20 fat bombs |

Ingredients:

- 1/2 cup sugar-free dark chocolate chips
- 3 cups almond flour
- 1/2 teaspoon sea salt
- 3/4 cup coconut oil
- 1 1/2 teaspoons vanilla extract
- 12-15 drops liquid stevia

For the coating:

- A few drops Easter themed natural food coloring
- 3/4 cup coconut butter, melted

Instructions:

1. Line a large baking sheet with parchment paper.
2. Add almond flour, coconut oil, vanilla extract, stevia and salt to a food processor. Pulse until it is well combined. Transfer into a bowl.
3. Add chocolate chips and fold gently.
4. Divide the mixture into 20 portions. Shape each portion into an egg using your hands. Place on the baking sheet.
5. Place the baking sheet in the freezer and chill until hardened.
6. Meanwhile, make the coating as follows: Divide the melted butter into 2 bowls.
7. To one bowl, add a few drops of food color and leave the other bowl as it is.

8. Dip one side of each of the eggs in the plain bowl and place on another lined baking sheet.
9. Add the colored butter to a zip lock bag. Cut off a little of the tip of the zip lock bag and pipe on the other part of the eggs.
10. Chill for an hour and serve. Unused ones can be frozen up to a month.

Coconut and Cinnamon Fat Bombs

Prep: 5 min	Total: 10 min + chilling time	Serving: 20 fat bombs

Ingredients:

- 2 cups canned, full fat coconut milk
- 2 cups finely shredded coconut
- 2 cups coconut butter or almond butter
- 1 teaspoon ground cinnamon
- 1 teaspoon ground nutmeg
- Erythritol or stevia to taste
- 2 teaspoons vanilla extract

Instructions:

1. Add all the ingredients (except shredded coconut) to a heatproof bowl.

2. Place the bowl in a double boiler. Heat until the mixture is well combined.
3. Remove from heat and chill for about 30 minutes or until it is soft enough to shape into balls.
4. Divide the mixture into 20 portions. Shape each into a ball. Dredge the balls in shredded coconut.
5. Place on a lined baking sheet.
6. Chill until it hardens and serve.

Vanilla Fat Bomb

Prep: 5 min	Total: 10 min + chilling time	Serving: 12 fat bombs

Ingredients:

- 16 ounces' cream cheese, warmed
- A pinch salt
- 1 cup erythritol or Swerve sweetener
- 1 cup heavy whipping cream
- 2 teaspoons vanilla extract
- 1 teaspoon sesame seeds
- 1 teaspoon poppy seeds

Instructions:

1. Add all the ingredients except whipping cream to a food processor. Set on medium speed.
2. While the food processor is operating, slowly drizzle the cream into it and blend until creamy.
3. Transfer into silicone moulds.
4. Dredge the balls in the coating mixture and place in an airtight container.
5. Chill and serve later.

Fudgy Macadamia Chocolate Fat Bombs

Prep: 5 min	Total: 10 min + chilling time	Serving: 12 fat bombs

Ingredients:

- 8 ounces' macadamia nuts, chopped
- 4 ounces' cocoa butter
- 4 tablespoons Swerve or erythritol
- 4 tablespoons cocoa, unsweetened
- 1/2 cup heavy cream or coconut oil

Instructions:

1. Add cocoa butter to a heatproof bowl.
2. Place the bowl in a double boiler. Heat until melted. Add cocoa and sweetener and stir until well combined.

3. Remove from heat and add macadamia nuts and stir.
4. Add cream and mix well.
5. Pour into silicone moulds and chill for about 30 minutes or until it hardens and serve.

Cinnamon Bun Fat Bomb Bars

Prep: 5 min	Total: 10 min + chilling time	Serving: 4 big bars

Ingredients:

- 1/4 teaspoon ground cinnamon
- 1 cup creamed coconut, chopped into chunks

For the first icing:

- 2 tablespoons almond butter
- 2 tablespoons extra virgin coconut oil, hardened

For the second icing:

- 1 teaspoon ground cinnamon
- 2 tablespoons almond butter

Instructions:

1. Add coconut cream and cinnamon to a bowl. Mix well using your hands. Transfer into a lined loaf pan.
2. To make the first icing: Add coconut oil and almond butter to a pan and whisk well.
3. Layer this over the coconut cream mixture in the loaf pan. Freeze for around 10 minutes.
4. Meanwhile, whisk together almond butter and cinnamon until smooth.
5. Layer this over the first icing.
6. Freeze for some more time.
7. Slice and serve.

Chocolate Raspberry Fat Bombs

Prep: 5 min	Total: 10 min + chilling time	Serving: 12

Ingredients:

- 6 tablespoons coconut oil
- 10 tablespoons butter
- 4 tablespoons sugar-free raspberry syrup
- 4 tablespoons cocoa powder

Instructions:

1. Add all the ingredients to a saucepan and place the saucepan over low heat.
2. Heat until the ingredients and melted.
3. Remove from heat. Cool slightly.
4. Pour into moulds.

5. Freeze and serve.

Chocolate Almond Fat Bomb

Prep: 5 min	Total: 10 min + chilling time	Serving: 18

Ingredients:

- ¾ cup coconut oil
- ¾ cup almond butter
- 5 tablespoons heavy whipping cream
- 4 ½ tablespoons cocoa, unsweetened
- 1 teaspoon vanilla extract
- 3 tablespoons erythritol or Swerve sweetener
- A pinch of salt
- ¼ choco chips

Instructions:

1. Place a saucepan over low heat. Add almond butter and coconut oil. Heat until melted.
2. Add the remaining ingredients and stir.
3. Remove from heat and pour into cupcake tin that is lined with cupcake papers.
4. Garnish with choco chips
5. Freeze for about 15-20 minutes or until hard.

Stacked Choco-nut Bombs

Prep: 5 min	Total: 15 min + chilling time	Serving: 18

Ingredients:

- 1 ¼ cups coconut oil, melted
- 1/3 cup peanut butter
- 1/3 cup cocoa powder, unsweetened
- Liquid Splenda to taste
- Nuts of your choice for garnish

Instructions:

1. Divide the melted coconut oil into 3 bowls.
2. In the first bowl, add cocoa powder and a little Splenda to it and stir.

3. To the second bowl, add peanut butter and a little Splenda and stir.
4. To the third bowl, add a little Splenda and stir.
5. Take 18 small muffin cups. Divide and spoon in the chocolate mixture into the muffin cups.
6. Chill until it is set.
7. Next spoon in the peanut butter mixture over the chocolate layer. Chill again in the refrigerator until set.
8. Next spoon in the Splenda mixture over the chocolate layer.
9. Chill again until set.

Chocolate Fat Bombs

| Prep: 5 min | Total: 15 min + freezing time | Serving: 10 |

Ingredients:

- 1/4 cup coconut oil
- 1/4 cup peanut butter
- 1/4 cup butter
- 1/2 cup dark chocolate chips, unsweetened

Instructions:

1. Add all the ingredients to a microwave safe bowl.
2. Microwave until the mixture melts. Stir a couple of times while it is melting.
3. Pour the mixture into ice cube trays.
4. Freeze and serve.

Valentine Day Treat

Prep: 2 min	Total: 7 min + freezing time	Serving: 8

Ingredients:

- 4 ounces' almond butter
- 4 ounces' coconut oil
- 1-ounce sugar-free vanilla syrup
- 2 ounces' cream cheese
- 4 ounces 85 % dark chocolate
- 2 teaspoons cocoa powder
- 12-15 drops stevia

Instructions:

1. Add all the ingredients except almond butter to a microwave safe container.

2. Microwave for 30 seconds and mix. Microwave for a few more seconds if the chocolate is not melted well.
3. Pour half the mixture into 8 silicone moulds.
4. Add a blob of almond butter in the center of each mould.
5. Pour the remaining mixture over it.
6. Freeze until set.
7. Remove from the freezer and place in the refrigerator until you serve.

Coconut Chocolate Fat Bombs

Prep: 5 min	Total: 20 min + freezing time	Serving: 20 fat bombs

Ingredients:

- 2 cups canned, full fat coconut milk
- 2 cups finely shredded coconut
- 2 cups coconut butter or almond butter
- 4 tablespoons cocoa powder, unsweetened
- Erythritol or stevia to taste
- 2 teaspoons vanilla extract
- 8 drops peppermint extract (optional)

Instructions:

1. Add all the ingredients except shredded coconut to a heatproof bowl.

2. Place the bowl in a double boiler. Heat until the mixture is well combined.
3. Remove from heat and chill for about 30 minutes or until it is soft enough to shape into balls.
4. Divide the mixture into 20 portions. Shape each into a ball. Dredge the balls in shredded coconut.
5. Place on a lined baking sheet.
6. Chill until it hardens and serve.

Easy Lemon Fat Bombs

Prep: 5 min	Total: 15 min + freezing time	Serving: 5

Ingredients:

- 2 tablespoons extra virgin coconut oil, softened, at room temperature
- 3.5 ounces' coconut butter, softened, at room temperature
- 10 drops stevia or to taste or 2 tablespoons erythritol
- 1 tablespoon lemon juice
- 1 teaspoon lemon zest, grated
- A pinch pink Himalayan salt

Instructions:

1. Mix together all the ingredients. Pour into silicone candy moulds or any other moulds you desire.
2. Chill until hardened.
3. Refrigerate until you serve.

Caramel Apple Pie Fat Bomb

| Prep: 5 min | Total: 10 min + freezing time | Serving: 16 |

Ingredients:

- 2 cans (5.4 ounces each) coconut cream
- 4 tablespoons coconut oil
- 1 cup coconut butter
- 4 medium green apples, peeled, cored, sliced
- 2 teaspoons ground cinnamon
- 40 drops English toffee stevia
- A large pinch sea salt

Instructions:

1. Place a skillet over medium heat. Add coconut oil. Add apples and cook until soft.
2. Add cinnamon and mix well.
3. Remove from heat and cool slightly.
4. Add to a blender along with the rest of the ingredients.
5. Pour into 16 small silicone muffin moulds.
6. Freeze and serve.

Pumpkin Pie Fat Bombs

Prep: 5 min	Total: 10 min + freezing time	Serving: 12

Ingredients:

- 1 cup long shredded coconut, unsweetened
- 2 tablespoons grass fed collagen
- 1/4 cup coconut oil
- 6 tablespoons pumpkin puree, unsweetened, warm
- 1/8 teaspoons pink Himalayan rock salt
- 3/4 teaspoon ground ginger
- 1/2 tablespoon ground cinnamon
- A pinch ground cloves
- 1/4 teaspoon vanilla extract
- 10-12 drops stevia

Instructions:

1. Place a 12-count silicone muffin moulds on a baking sheet.
2. Add coconut, coconut oil, stevia and salt to a food processor and blend until smooth.
3. Remove about 1/4 of the blended mixture from the blender and set aside.
4. Add the remaining ingredients to the blender and blend until smooth.
5. Remove from the blender and transfer into the silicone muffin moulds. Press it slightly so that it settles at the bottom.
6. Spoon in the mixture that was set aside on top of the pumpkin mixture.
7. Place the baking sheet in the freezer and freeze until hard.

Orange & Walnut Chocolate Fat Bombs

Prep: 5 min	Total: 15 min + chilling time	Serving: 10

Ingredients:

- 2.2 ounces 85% dark chocolate
- 2/3 cup walnuts, chopped
- 2 tablespoons extra virgin olive oil
- 1/2 teaspoon ground cinnamon
- 1 teaspoon fresh orange peel, finely chopped
- 1/2 teaspoon orange extract
- 8 drops stevia or any sweetener of your choice

Instructions:

1. Place chocolate, coconut oil and cinnamon in a heatproof bowl. Place the bowl in a double boiler.
2. Heat until the chocolate melts.
3. Add stevia and mix well. Remove from heat.
4. Add walnuts, orange extract, and orange peel and mix well.
5. Pour into candy cups or in the shape you desire
6. Chill until it is hard.

Keto Mounds Fat Bombs

| Prep: 5 min | Total: 15 min + chilling time | Serving: 12 |

Ingredients:

For the balls:

- 1 cup shredded coconut, unsweetened
- 2 tablespoons butter, melted
- 2 tablespoons coconut oil
- Stevia to taste
- 1/4 teaspoon vanilla extract

For the coating:

- 1/2 cup dark chocolate, unsweetened
- Stevia drops to taste
- 2 tablespoons coconut oil

Instructions:

1. To make the balls: Add all the ingredients of the ball to a food processor and blend until smooth.
2. Place in the refrigerator for about 15 minutes or until slightly set.
3. Make 1-inch balls of the mixture and place on a lined baking sheet.
4. Refrigerate for an hour.
5. Place a saucepan over low heat. Add chocolate and heat until it melts.
6. Add coconut oil and sweetener and stir. Remove from heat and cool for 5 minutes.
7. Remove the chilled balls from the refrigerator and dip into the chocolate mixture. Place on the baking sheet.
8. Freeze and serve later.

Orange Butter Pecan Fat Bombs

Prep: 5 min	Total: 15 min + chilling time	Serving: 12

Ingredients:

- 24 pecan halves, toasted
- 3 teaspoons orange zest, finely grated
- 3 tablespoons butter, unsalted, softened
- A pinch sea salt

Instructions:

1. Add butter and orange zest to a bowl and stir.
2. Place 12 pecan halves on a baking sheet. Divide and spread the butter mixture over it.
3. Cover with the other half.
4. Chill in the refrigerator for an hour and serve.

Conclusion

Thank you once again for downloading this book. Initially you might have thought that implementing the Ketogenic diet is a mountain to climb. In fact, it isn't. It's a very simple diet and you needn't cut corners when it comes to your diet. You will just have to limit the carbs that you are consuming. You can eat your favorite sweet treats without putting on any extra weight and you will actually start to lose weight in this process. Eating fat to lose fat definitely works. If you don't believe it, the only way in which you can change your opinion is by trying it once. I am sure the results will definitely convince you to opt for the Ketogenic lifestyle.

If you are serious about following your diet, then you can maintain a food journal where you write down about everything that you have been consuming and your body measurements and weight as well. After a few weeks on this diet you will definitely see a positive change. The recipes given in this book are not only good for you but you wouldn't feel guilty after consuming them. They taste as good as, if not better than the actual treats that you are used to gorging on. You can tweak the recipes slightly to suit your needs.

So, get started right now. It is not that difficult, a little bit of effort can work wonders for you! So get going and all the best!

All the best!

www.ingramcontent.com/pod-product-compliance
Lightning Source LLC
Chambersburg PA
CBHW070944080526
44587CB00015B/2220